# Eek! My Mummy
# Has Breast Cancer
# by Emma Sutherland

~Eek! My Mummy Has Breast Cancer~

*It is important to do your own self-awareness checks and if you find something not 'normal' please do consult your doctor*

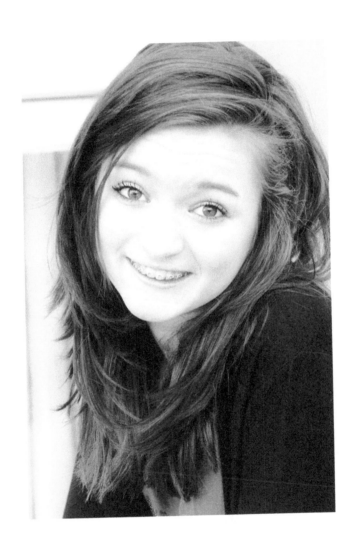

# Hi, I'm Emma

First published in the United Kingdom 2013.
Copyright © Emma Sutherland  All rights reserved.

© Artwork by Leanne Hamilton
© Photos by Dot McQueen
© Polaroid Image by Opicobello
© Pink Ribbon Image by Koya979
© Cover Design  by Plan4 Media

A catalogue record of this book is available from the British Library.

ISBN 978-1-907463-78-5

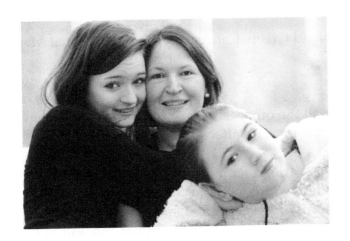

Eek! My Mummy Has Breast Cancer:
*Our journey - two girls' story*

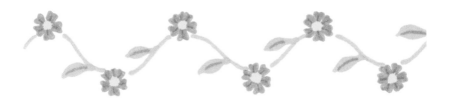

# Dedication

To Professor Mike Dixon, Consultant Surgeon, Edinburgh's
Western General
– for saving my mummy.

To Seonaid Green, Cancer Support Specialist at Maggie's
Edinburgh
– for saving Me.

And for all the other teenage boys and girls who have been
affected by cancer.

To my best friend Jenny Mulhern and her family for their
incredibly kind donation. To my BMBFFAAT, and the
Mulherns; the best second family ever. Their donation
enabled me to give Maggie's Edinburgh and Maggie's
Glasgow 100 books each.

...and to you, for buying my book

**Love Emma xxxxx**

Hi, my name is Emma. I'm 12 and I live with my mum, Rosie (41) and sister Kate (9). We have a happy life, do normal things like school, work, eat and drink and meet with friends. My mum is funny. She makes us laugh lots and is always there for us. It's funny how you live your life not knowing what's round the corner.

One Friday afternoon, 3rd February 2012 to be exact, my sister and I came home from dancing when Mum shouted us through to the living-room for a *Newsflash*. Newflash in our house means that something exciting is about to happen like a holiday to Florida! My sister and I sat on the settee in our ordinary living-room in our ordinary house on an ordinary day.

"I don't want you to get upset or worry," said my mum. At that point I didn't know what was coming but it wasn't a holiday! I took the cushion that was next to me and slowly pulled it to cover my face. That way no one would see me cry. "A few weeks ago I found a lump in my right boob. I went to the doctors and they sent me to the hospital for a check up. So...I'm just back from the hospital today and I was told that I have breast cancer." *WOOOOSH!* My head was spinning.

**Breast Cancer Statistic**

**55,000 people are diagnosed with breast cancer every year**

Is this actually happening? I thought. What? WHAT? I was confused. My mum doesn't get cancer. It happens to other people. Cancer?

As my sister and I sat listening to my mum I felt every emotion inside me drain away. I was numb.

My mum went on to say that there was a wee lump that had to be removed with a small operation.

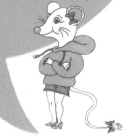

## Lumpectomy

Usually when someone has breast cancer a surgeon will operate and remove the tumour. Sometimes the surgeon will be able to remove just the tumour and a little bit of the normal tissue around the lump. This is called a lumpectomy. Sometimes the surgeon will need to take away the whole breast instead of just the lump, and this is called a mastectomy.

## Lumpectomy

Usually the surgery is carried out by a specialist breast surgeon, who is very experienced in these types of operation, and because the breast is not deep within the body it is fairly straightforward surgery. People usually recover quickly from the surgery and can be back at home within a few days.

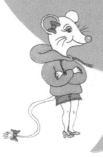

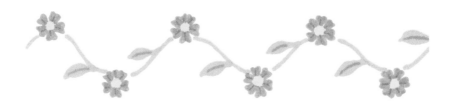

Then she would go on to get radiotherapy. My mum tried to make us laugh by saying she was going to wear a bikini and pretend she was in Barbados. I didn't really find it funny as I didn't know what radiotherapy was.

I do remember one thing clearly. At the end my mum said that her doctor told her it was not life threatening. I didn't believe her. People who get cancer usually die...or so I thought.

# Radiotherapy

Radiotherapy is used to treat lots of different kinds of cancer, and most people who have breast cancer will have radiotherapy treatment. Radiotherapy is treatment using X-Rays, and people having treatment will feel nothing. It's like going for a normal X-Ray, except the X-Rays have more energy and so can be used to damage and kill any cancer cells which have been left behind after the surgery. Sometimes people will have Radiotherapy treatment before their surgery, and this helps to shrink the tumour so that less tissue has to be removed during surgery. This is very helpful for larger tumours. Most people will have their radiotherapy after their surgery.

# Radiotherapy

The radiotherapy will kill cancer cells, because cancer cells have lost the ability to recover if they are damaged. It will also cause some damage to healthy cells, but the dose given will allow the healthy cells to repair and recover after the treatment has finished. The treatment is very focused and can be aimed very accurately at the area where the cancer grew within the breast.

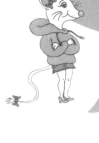

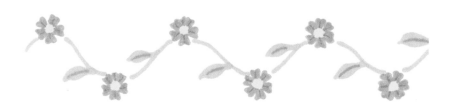

## Radiotherapy

None of the rest of the body will be treated, and because the treatment uses X-Rays there is no radiation once the treatment machine has been turned off. This means that it's perfectly safe to be around someone who is having radiotherapy treatment.
Radiotherapy can make the skin of the area having treatment turn quite pink. This can look and feel a bit like mild sunburn

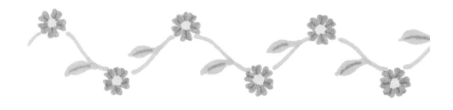

Hindsight is a wonderful thing and I can see now how uneducated I was about cancer. But who reads about it when it's not part of your life?

"Any questions?" my mum asked. Kate, who sat still throughout, probably not really understanding what had just been said, asked, "Yes, can I go back to the computer now?" This made me giggle inside but not enough to show on my face. I just asked to go to my room and I ran upstairs as quickly as I could and buried my face in my pillow and cried like I had never cried before.

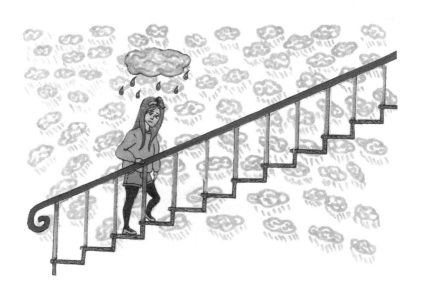

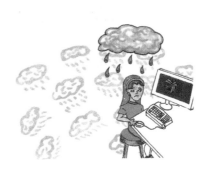

I phoned my friend. My mum had already told my friend's mum just a few hours earlier as she knew I would want to speak to Jenny. Jenny had lost a friend to breast cancer and I felt she was the right person to support me. We talked on the phone for an hour – well I just sobbed and listened.

After I put the phone down my mum came into my room. She could see I had been sobbing as my mascara was all over my bed sheets, not to mention my face! We hugged and cried together as I wondered if she was going to be ok.

My mum is my rock. She guides me, keeps me safe, gives me pocket money and makes me eat green beans! She is such a loving caring fun mum – I can't ever imagine my life without her. She had lots of biopsies done, she was very sore.

That whole weekend was a bit of a blur. Mum had a lot of biopsies done and was very sore, but we still managed a nice walk.

**Why we need biopsies and what they prove**
Whenever the doctors think that someone has cancer they will take a small sample of the tumour. This sample is called a biopsy, and for breast cancer it is taken using a needle which is pushed through the skin into the lump. The tissue sample is then sent off to the labs, where it is looked at under a microscope. By examining the cells from the biopsy, the doctors can tell whether the lump in the breast is actually cancer or not.

Over the next few weeks my mum needed even more biopsies as her diagnosis changed.

**Why we need biopsies and what they prove**

If it is cancer, they can also find out lots of useful information about what type of breast cancer the person has, and the way that these particular cancer cells behave. All this information is used to grade the tumour, and this helps the doctors decide which treatments to use to treat the cancer.

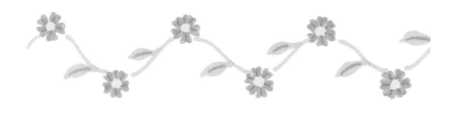

She would always go to the Western General Hospital on a Tuesday. The news seemed to be getting worse. The next again visit they confirmed that the cancer was bigger than they originally thought so another set of biopsies were required. It wasn't nice seeing the bruising on my mum's breast. I wanted to help and make it all better but I just felt helpless.

I wanted to ask questions but I was afraid I would make my mum upset as the last thing she probably wanted to talk about was cancer. So I didn't ask. Nobody told me any real details so I turned to the internet. Wow! if you type in "Breast Cancer" a zillion websites come up. Some of them are quite scary and a lot of them talk about death but not too many were for teenagers, people my age, in words I could understand. I was confused by all the big words and ifs and buts. I needed to know my mum was going to be ok but even the doctors couldn't confirm this yet as the final diagnosis was still to be made.

A few weeks passed and my mum sat us down again. What on earth was she going to say to us this time?

"Ok...remember I told you I needed a lumpectomy and radiotherapy? Well things have changed a little. I need to get my whole breast removed. The cancer has spread – the doctor explained it to me like a bomb of cancer cells exploding in my breast. So we need to get rid of the cancer and that is my only option. I don't have a date for my operation yet – it may be in May sometime".

I couldn't believe it. My mum was now going to lose a breast!

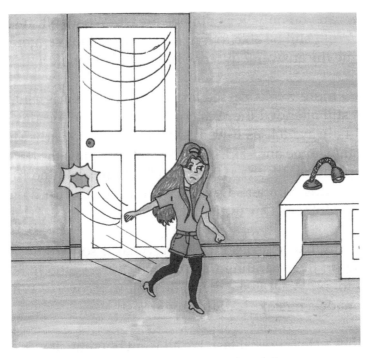

I was very angry. Why us?

## Mastectomy

Mastectomy is the removal of a whole breast, and is the surgery which is chosen if there are a few different lumps, or areas of cancer in the breast. It is also sometimes used if the lump is very big.

How can you only live with one breast? What will she look like? Will I still be able to hug my mum? Who was going to give me the answers? No-one so I just kept quiet.

A few more weeks passed and nothing more was said. My mum still attended the Western General every Tuesday and would always tell us it went well. However in early March she came home and said, "That's it then – I have the date for my operation. It's the 19th March." Oh my goodness... it's the day after Mother's Day. I HAVE to make this the most special Mother's Day ever.

Then my real worries kicked in. What if something went wrong on the operating table? What if it was too hard for them to fix? What if she didn't do well in recovery? What if they made a mistake? All these worries!

Mother's Day came at last. We all went bowling. It was such fun and I actually forgot my mum was going into hospital at 7am the next day. We bought a Mother's Day helium balloon and mum decided it was going into hospital with her the next day. My mum was her usual self and we laughed, joked, played pool and even went to the Stable Bar for some lunch. Our little life seemed so normal to everyone around us. We were a normal family having a normal day.

Monday 19th March 2012: I got up for school and my mum was already up. She said she was so hungry but wasn't allowed to eat anything as she was having her operation that day. It seemed like a normal morning. It came to 7.30am and time for me to leave for the bus. My mum didn't seem any different but I now know she was terrified that morning but didn't want to show her emotions. We actually walked down the street together – I went for my bus and my mum went to her friend's house a few doors down who was taking her to the hospital. I continued down the street with my ear phones in listening to music. My favourite track at the time was 'Beautiful' by Christina Aguilera. Seems quite appropriate now. I somehow managed to keep it all altogether until I got on my school bus. I sat down and cried. I was on the bus alone with my tears, my thoughts and missing my mummy already.

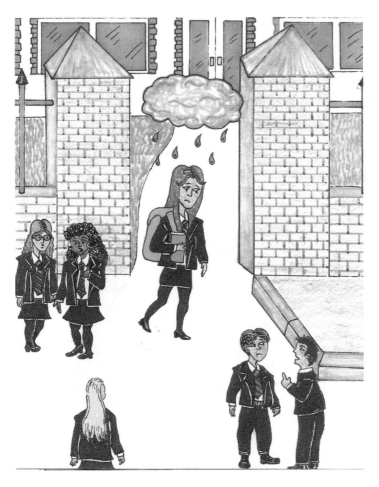

I so often felt alone and completely isolated. School was dreadful for me during this time as it seemed everyone was living in another world from me; the world I wanted to be in - just to be a normal teenager.

It was a very long day at school. I was told that I could come out of class whenever I wanted to (if I needed to). I didn't though as I didn't want to lose it in front of my friends. I was trying to remain strong. Eventually the 3.30pm school bell rang – thank goodness. My mum had arranged for me to go back to my friend Jenny's house. She was the friend that listened to me crying the day my mum was diagnosed so I knew I was in good hands. We had dinner and didn't talk about the operation at all. I actually did German revision as we had a test the next day. During my German revision I got a phone call – from the hospital! It was my mum. She started talking about hunting? Ha Ha! She was just out of recovery and still full of anaesthetic. To this day my mum can't remember talking to me or my sister.

I was excited just to hear my mum's voice and that she was out of the operating theatre. I was going to visit her the next again day at the hospital.

## Recovery

Recovery is the area next to an operating theatre where people will be taken as soon as their surgery is finished. When they are wheeled into recovery they will still be anesthetised, but this will slowly wear off and they will wake up. They are watched closely here and their heart rate and other vital functions are monitored. Once the nurses in recovery are happy that the person is fully awake and recovered from the anaesthetic they will have them transferred back to the ward.

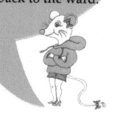

Kate and I arrived at the hospital with various bits and pieces for my mum. We didn't know what room she was in. I started to get scared and my breathing got faster. I remember standing outside when the nurse told us what room my mum was in. We walked in and saw Mum lying on the hospital bed. She was full of drips and drains and looked grey. She still had her hospital gown on – I seriously didn't recognise my fun-loving mum. I couldn't go near her. I couldn't cuddle her. I couldn't get to her for all the equipment. It was scary and upsetting. We sat down to watch the TV to take our mind off how my mum looked because she wasn't very well at all. The nurses ended up coming to take care of her as she was really ill.

## Explaining Noises
## & Smells  et cetera...

When somebody has had surgery they will often have some drains, which are tubes coming out of the body, about the width of a straw. A drain allows fluid from the operation site to drain quickly out of the body into a bag which hangs down below the bed. It speeds up the healing process and reduces the risk of an infection. Usually they will also have an IV drip, which hangs above the bed and allows fluids and painkillers to be given easily and over a period of time, directly into the veins.

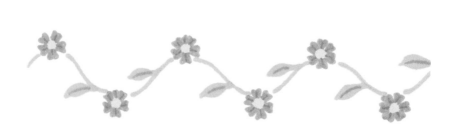

**Explaining Noises**
**& Smells  et cetera...**

This is the most effective way to deliver medication, without the person having to swallow lots of tablets. Usually after surgery the nurses will also attach a finger clip, which looks like a giant clothes peg, so that the level of oxygen in the blood, the blood pressure and their heart rate can all be measured. There will be a digital display screen showing all of these measurements beside the bed. Sometimes the sound on the monitor will be turned up and this will beep to help the nurses keep an eye on what's happening.

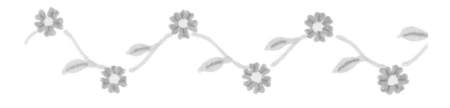

### Why was Mum ill?

After surgery people can have all sorts of reactions to the anaesthetic drugs, and to the pain killers. Most people recover quickly but some people can have bad reactions, like sickness, or low blood pressure. Usually it's the first time that people have taken the medications which are used for surgery, and so the doctors and nurses can't be sure how someone's body will react. This is one of the reasons they keep such a close eye on people after surgery. Until these drugs are out of their body people can feel and look very unwell.

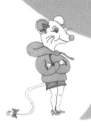

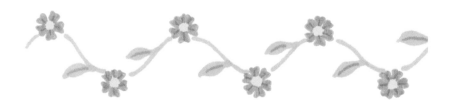

I didn't want to leave but at the same time I couldn't stay in that room any longer. I was too upset. The minute we left the room my sister and I both burst into tears. This strong woman who has taken care of us looked frail and weak.

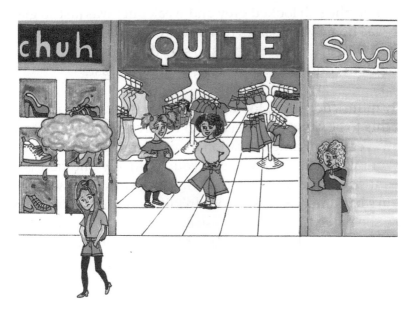

I feel sad and confused

I didn't want to go back and visit my mum. Not because I didn't want to see her but hospitals are scary especially when it's a close relative and they have things attached to them that you have never seen before. I have only ever seen this kind of stuff on the television.

So I continued to stay with friends and went to school as normal. My amazing friends kept my mind busy with other things and life went on as normal. I didn't see my mum at all that week but on Friday afternoon I got a call on my mobile. I was at the park with friends. It was my mum! She was phoning to tell me that she was allowed to come home – YEE HA! Was this for real? It was too soon!    Quick – off to the number 11 bus stop I go! By the time I get the bus home from the park my mum would be home.

I got home to see my mum lying on the couch with a blanket over her. She still looked grey and weak but I was just so glad she was home with us. It's really weird for me to only see my mum twice in a week. She was so sore that I couldn't get close enough to cuddle her. How long would this last?

My mum's operation took the cancer cells away but in order for this to be done they needed to remove her whole breast. However in the same operation they were able to reconstruct my mum's boob so I suppose you could say she had two operations. The surgeon did the reconstruction with my mum's back muscle so she couldn't lift and she had to watch how she moved. She couldn't sleep properly as she had a big wound on her back and her front was sore due to the operation.

**Facts on reconstruction**

Following a mastectomy many people will chose to have a breast rebuilt, to look the same as it did before. If the type of cancer, and the surgery means that they will not need radiotherapy treatment, then this reconstruction can be done immediately after the breast has been removed. This means that they will only need to be anaesthetised once.

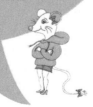

Over the next few weeks my sister and I became my mum's carers. We made her cups of tea and plates of toast, helped her get dressed, helped her up off the settee – basically did everything for her as she couldn't do a thing for herself. I hadn't realised how incapacitated my mum would be but I was determined not to let her lift a thing. My mum couldn't drive so we relied on family and friends to help us get where we needed to be, to bring in shopping and to take us to dancing class. Mum was trying to make our life seem normal but all I could see was a mum that couldn't even stretch for a cup.

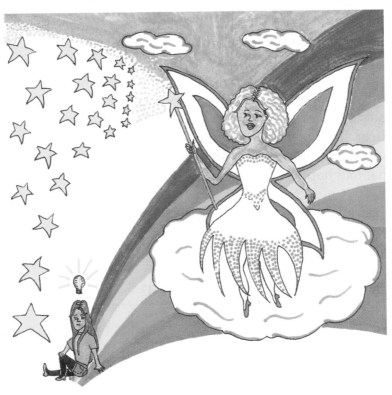

We needed a fairy godmother

Over the next few weeks my mum gradually got a wee bit stronger and was able to do a little more for herself and us but all I did was continually worry. I worried when I saw her pick up a heavy milk carton from the fridge, or when she stretched for the cereal. I didn't want my mum to do anything – I wanted to do it all. My worrying got the better of me and I didn't manage my feelings well.

By the time my mum was better and 80% back to normal we were having to deal with my issue of not coping with my mum having cancer. I think I was a bit numb to be honest. I didn't talk to anyone really as I didn't want to. I didn't know where to turn. I ended up speaking to a Cancer Support Specialist at Maggie's Centre. They had worked in the hospital for years talking to people with cancer, and so they were able to explain what had happened to my mum and why. They also helped me talk about how scared I was, but made me feel totally normal, as everyone gets scared of cancer. It was like someone turning on the light. With knowledge comes power and I had the power to understand what had happened to our family.

I had all these questions:

What is cancer?

I thought if you had cancer you died?

Would the cancer come back?

Will my mum ever fully recover?

Would I get breast cancer?

Why didn't my mum need chemotherapy or radiotherapy?

My constant worry was my mum wasn't telling me the truth but now I was armed with the facts I felt a lot better about the whole situation. I started to relax and didn't panic as much when my mum went to lift a bag.

My family had no history of cancer and this was a real shock to all of us. My Nana was in shock, my aunties were in shock and we were definitely in shock.

However It's really important you know that every cancer is different. There are good stories and some not so good stories. There are people who lose their hair and people who don't! People who need their boobs removed and people who only need a lumpectomy.

**It's important to talk about your feelings**

You can talk to someone you trust, write it down, exercise, which can release frustration, or have a good cry as tears contain chemicals that can build up and cause tension. You want to avoid having negative thoughts which can happen when you are scared or confused. Showing and managing your feelings allows you to let off steam slowly rather than exploding.

## Chemotherapy

Lots of people who have breast cancer will need radiotherapy as well as surgery, and some people will also need chemotherapy.

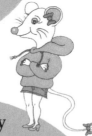

## Chemotherapy

Chemotherapy is treatment using drugs which are toxic to the cancer cells. It is usually a fluid given through an IV drip, which means that it goes into a vein and is then pumped around the body by the heart. This means that the person's whole body will be treated. It's used if the doctors think there's a risk that some cancer cells might have travelled away from the original lump, and moved to other places in the body.

## Chemotherapy

Chemotherapy for breast cancer is usually given every three weeks, and the doctor will normally prescribe six to eight treatments. Each treatment is called a cycle, and people need to have a blood test done to check that their white blood cells have recovered enough, before the next dose will be given.

## Chemotherapy

White blood cells are what the body's immune system is made up of, and so during part of their treatment cycle people will have a reduced immune response. This means that someone on chemotherapy can pick up infections more easily, and so they may need to avoid places with big groups of people who might be carrying infections. They might also need to use a different towel in the bathroom at home, to help to keep infections away from them.

## Chemotherapy

Some of the drugs can make people feel tired much more quickly than usual, and some drugs can make people feel sick, as though they had constant travel sickness. This means that they might like different foods from normal, and they might even have some cravings for food they don't usually like.

## Chemotherapy

Some, but not all, chemotherapy drugs will affect the cells at the roots of the hair, and this causes peoples hair to fall out. Most of the chemotherapy drugs used to treat breast cancer will affect the hair roots, and so cause hair loss, not just head hair, but all body hair including eyebrows and eyelashes. Once they have finished their treatment their hair will grow back in again, but it can take several months before this happens.

## Chemotherapy

All of these side effects are temporary. It's important to remember that it's the chemotherapy treatments and not the cancer which makes people feel unwell during treatment.

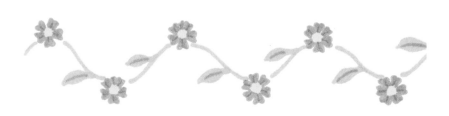

We thought Maggie's Centres were for old people who were going to die! They are not! Also family and friends are welcome – it's not just cancer sufferers. Maggie's is the most amazing inspirational bright positive place to go and meet the most amazing people who have incredible knowledge of what you are going through. They are very kind and sincere and you are always welcome for refreshments.

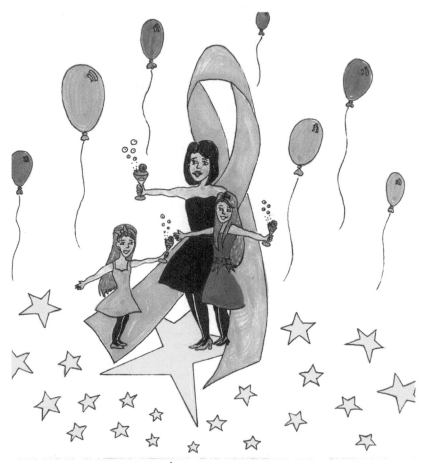

Finally in June my mum received the all clear. I was ecstatic. I couldn't believe it was all over – the cancer was gone. All my mum has to do is take one tablet every day for five years.

**Tamoxifen, Arimadex and Examesatone are the most commonly used medicines for hormone dependent breast cancers, and they are taken as one small daily tablet.**

### Tamoxifen

Taking these drugs can prevent cancer recurring by stopping them growing or thriving. It's a good 'just in case' treatment which usually doesn't cause too many side effects. The most common side effects are symptoms which are just like the menopause, because the hormonal environment in the body has been changed by the drugs.

Lots of people who have had breast cancer will be given hormonal treatment to take for a number of years. Not everyone needs this type of treatment, you only need it if the biopsy showed that there were oestrogen receptors on the original cancer cells. If the cancer cells had oestrogen receptors, then hormonal treatments will help to switch off or slow down any cancer cells which may have been left behind after treatment.

When I was told about my mum's diagnosis I shrieked *'Eek! My mummy has breast cancer'.*

I didn't know much about breast cancer but in a strange twist of fate I *had* to learn more about it for my own sake, and for the sake of other teenagers who might be going through the same thing as I did.

I wanted other teenagers to have information that was easier to understand from a teenager's point of view, and what better way to reach out to other teenagers than to have the information come from a teenager; a teenager who has been there and lived through those times with a parent who has been diagnosed with the dreaded disease.

I know there is a need for this book and if this book has helped someone else in some way, no matter how small, then this whole journey and project has been well worth it.

Thank you for reading my story.

*Emma x*

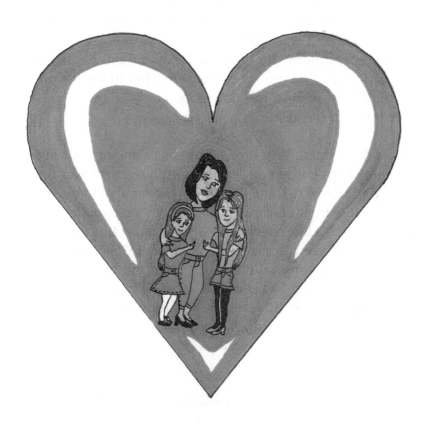

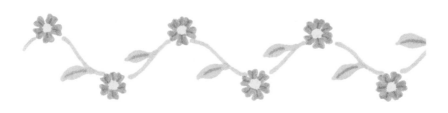

# Words From My Family

I remember the day Mum sat us down on the couch and told us she had breast cancer. I was very scared as I didn't know what this was. I had no clue what was going to happen next. My mummy wasn't crying so I knew that everything would be ok in the end. But when I saw my sister's reaction I was worried.

Seeing my mummy go through the operation was horrible and I cried the first time we went to see her in the hospital. Thankfully the cancer has now gone.
**Kate** *(my sister)* **Age 10**

I was devastated. Whatever happens to one of your family members happens to you. When I got the news it was one of shock and horror to think that one of the family members had fallen to the dreaded cancer. And there's no explanation for the feelings. It's like a feeling of loss, because this is a disease that's out of your control. Because there's so much of it around, you feeling you're falling into the black hole that you're never going to get out of. I felt helpless because you can't help them. Sometimes these things have to take their course and hope that things will sort itself out for the good, and if it does, then you're one of the lucky ones.
**My Nana (Irene)**

The day I got the call from my sister to say she had just been told she had invasive breast cancer, I was enjoying a drink in the pub with hubby James, catching up with the daily normal grind of work. I could not believe what I had been told. I was shocked and stunned and I just could not take it in. I came off the phone with Rosie and told James, "What? that can't be right!" he said. I don't think he could believe it either by that time I was already in tears! My sister Rosie had cancer! It can't be true, she is younger than me; such a young woman and we had no trace of cancer in the family. This was devastating news to the family and for Rosie and the girls *(Emma and Kate)*. However Rosie was made of something special, and had even more courage, strength and determination to battle this evil and win the battle, with help and support from friends and family. She was fighting not only for her own life but for that of Emma and Kate's too, and she won her battle. We are so proud of Rosie but also of Emma and Kate for helping their mum. **My Aunty Irene**

I remember Mum told me and I was shocked and devastated, because there was no history in the family of it. At the time I thought if I would change places with her I would, because she was so young and she had to go through this all on her own. It is a constant worry because she is going back to the hospital in March 2013 to make sure it's all away. **My Aunty Jane**

When Rosie first told me she found a lump I tried to think positively and reassured her that it was probably nothing. I was gutted when the worst was confirmed. As a friend of many years I felt helpless and wished I could take the pain and fear away from Rosie, Emma and Kate. I saw Rosie the day after she got out of hospital and was terrified of seeing her so ill. Despite everything Rosie kept her sense of humour, remained positive and an inspiration to all. I was so relieved when Rosie got the news that the op had been a success. I am so proud to call Rosie, Emma and Kate my friends. **Lynne Bannan xxx** *(my mum's friend of nearly 20 years)*

# Photo Gallery

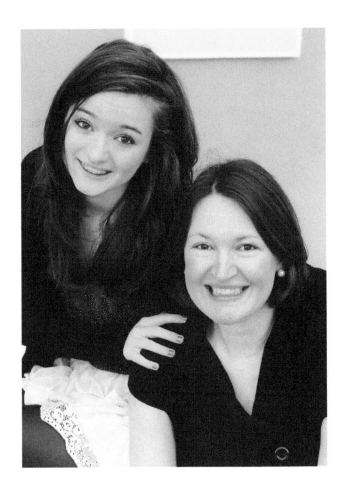

Emma & Mummy, Rosie

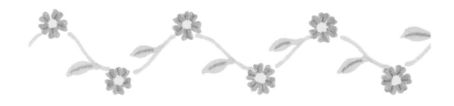

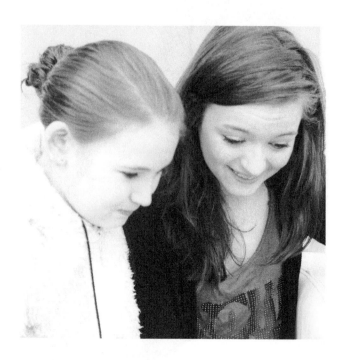

Emma & Kate

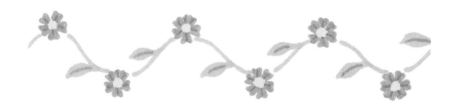

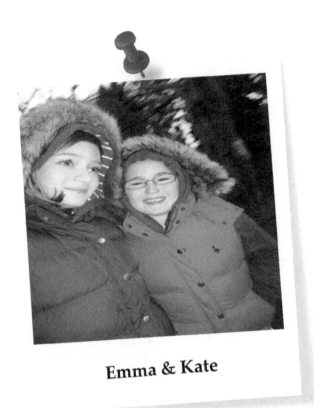

**Emma & Kate**

On a walk at Hermitage of Braid in Edinburgh.
Mum has just told us the news the day before.
We tried to remain positive.

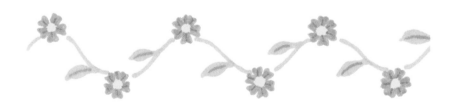

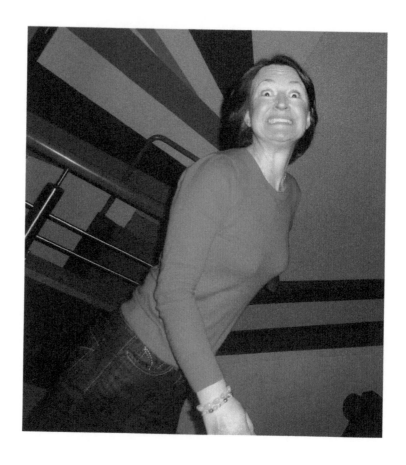

My mum the very day before her operation.
We went bowling. She tried to keep things as normal as
possible for us.

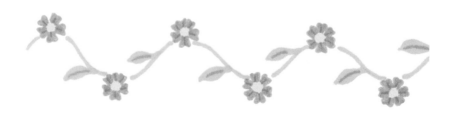

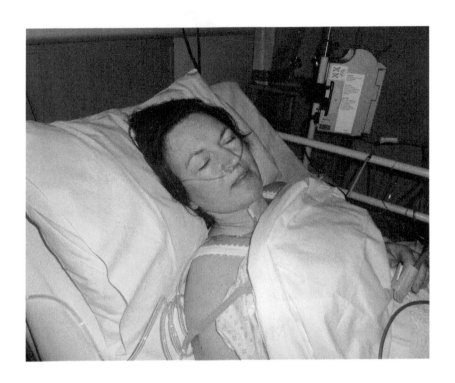

Our Mummy after her operation.

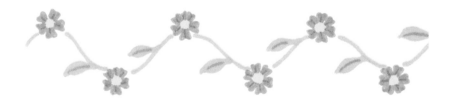

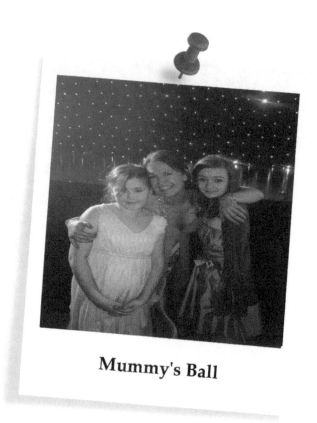

**Mummy's Ball**

My mummy, Kate and Me at "Mummy's Ball" which raised
£25,000 for Breast Cancer Care.
This was 8 weeks after my mum's operation.
She danced the night away with 350 other people.

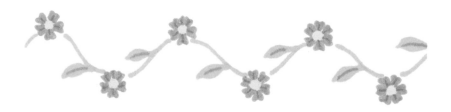

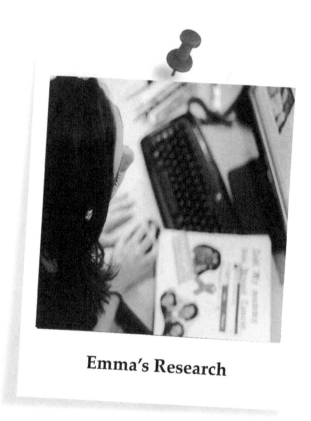

**Emma's Research**

This is me carrying out some research on breast cancer and gathering as much information as I can for the book. There is so much to learn about breast cancer.

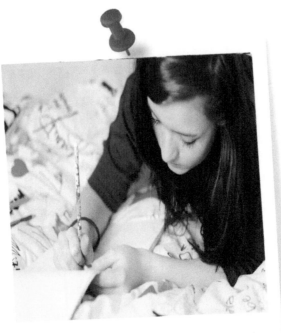

**Emma Working on Her Book**

Putting all the pieces together for
Eek! My Mummy Has Breast Cancer.

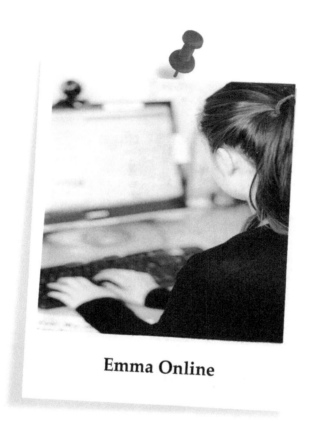

**Emma Online**

Here I am compiling all the gathered information into my computer where the files will be sent to the publisher for printing and distribution.

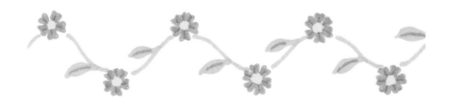

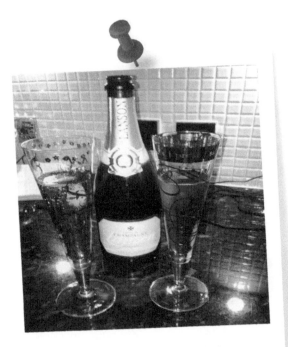

**Celebrating the all-clear**

As a family we go through everything together and given the all-clear meant we rightfully celebrated together.

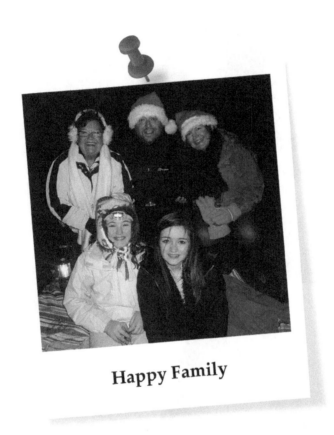

**Happy Family**

A happy family.
The end of our journey and year.
2013 is a new year - a very healthy happy one.

Nana, Scott, Rosie, Kate, and Emma

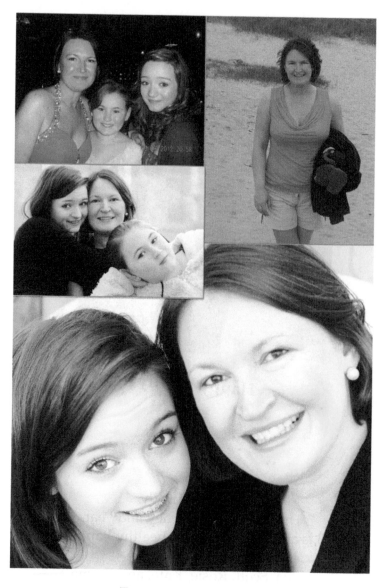

Emma, Kate & Rosie

# One Year On

It has now been nearly one year since our cancer journey began. My mum is doing really well and we are back to living our fun-filled happy life. We have been so lucky to come out the other end of this and say that we made it.

For me personally I have learned that it's nice to plan ahead but sometimes a little surprise along the way is not what you need. It doesn't mean you have to stop living; just appreciate your family, friends and loved ones more and everything they do for you. I would say that I am a typical teenager but instead of spending time in my room I spend time with my mum. We chat, laugh, cook and enjoy life.

The whole journey was a shock but we are stronger as a family and more grateful than ever to have our health.

We have raised a lot of money for various cancer charities since February 2012. I did a sponsored silence with my friend Jenny, Kate and I did the Race for Life, we helped my mum with a charity Ball which raised nearly £30,000. We will continue to give back as these amazing nurses, doctors, specialists and support network people at Maggie's have changed our lives forever.

# Cancer: the facts

C ancer can be a frightening word to hear, especially if you're hearing it because someone in your family has been diagnosed with it. It's important to remember that there are well over 300 types of cancer, and all of them will behave and be treated differently. Some cancers are much easier to treat than others, and breast cancer is one of the cancers that doctors are getting really good at treating. This means that more and more people are surviving and going on to live cancer-free lives after their treatment. Sometimes the doctors can't get rid of all the cancer, but scientists have created lots of new drugs which mean that cancer can be managed in the body. This means that people who have ongoing cancer, can usually live active lives with few side effects and lots of stretches of time where they feel well enough to do all the things they enjoy with their families.

Cancer is not usually something which happens because of anything someone has done or not done. It is something which happens because of a number of small changes deep within the nucleus of the cells in our bodies. Small flaws and changes happen naturally over time, and sometimes enough changes happen across a small area of DNA to result in cancerous changes to the cell. Changes in the cells can happen when the cells in our bodies divide. The older you are the higher the chances of cancer developing in your body, because your cells will have divided more often.

So you can see that cancer isn't something that you can catch, or something you can prevent happening. Sometimes people worry about the risk of passing cancer on to their children, so it's important to know that only a tiny percentage of cancer is inherited in the DNA. As an example, only 5% of breast cancers are thought to have a genetic basis, this means that 95% have no genetic basis. Normally families who carry a gene for cancer will be aware of this because there will be high numbers of family members who have developed cancer, usually at a fairly young age. If the doctors think there might be a genetic cause, they will ask some questions, before referring the person on for genetic testing.

Eating lots of healthy foods, and taking exercise will not stop anyone getting cancer, but it will mean that your body is in better shape to fight the cancer, and to recover from treatments. People sometimes feel angry if they have followed a healthy lifestyle, and they still get cancer, but again it's important to remember that taking care of your body is never wasted, as it means that your body has a head start in coping with treatment.

The Grade of a cancer is something which is discovered from the biopsy sample. It describes the nature and behaviour of the cells which make up the tumour. It helps the doctors understand the speed at which the cancer cells are likely to grow, and helps them chose the best treatment for those particular cells. Higher grade tumours grow faster than low grades, but the high grades also respond better to treatments like chemotherapy. The grade of someone's cancer is really only important for helping the doctors to pick the best treatments.

The stage of a cancer is like a map describing how much cancer there is, and where it is in the body. This also helps the doctors to prescribe the best treatment for the cancer which is present, and helps them predict where the cancer might go next, and so keeps everyone a step ahead of the tumour.

# maggie's
### People with cancer need places like these

Maggie's Centres provide free emotional, practical and social support to people with cancer and their families and friends, from Centres built in the grounds of specialist NHS cancer hospitals designed by leading architects. Whatever type of cancer you've got and whatever stage you're at, Maggie's is there to help and no appointments are necessary. The Centres are warm, friendly, informal places, full of light and open space and with a big kitchen at their heart. They provide a bridge from the stress of dealing with hospitals and treatment.

Maggie's also provides a peaceful space to absorb the information that you're inevitably bombarded with and helps to relieve some of the distress of having cancer. You can get the clarity you need from the professional experts who work at Maggie's. They'll listen to your questions or your concerns and provide the practical and emotional support and information to help you find your way through cancer.

The purpose of Maggie's is to help people who are feeling as if they've been kicked in the stomach by a cancer diagnosis to get on with their lives again. What they discover may help them put a different perspective on what is happening to them and make a profound difference to their experience of living with cancer.

# Facts and Talk about Teen Days and Days for Kids etc

Maggie's Centres in Edinburgh run Teen Days, for 12-19 year-olds who have a parent or significant family member with cancer. In Edinburgh we run two a year, always on a Saturday. The day includes a visit to the hospital where professional staff who treat people with cancer show us how and why they deliver the treatments. They also explain how the treatment works, and answer any questions about side effects. Often we will see behind the scenes to areas where the parent hasn't been, and there are lots of opportunities for hands on experience of all the high tech kit which is used.

Next comes lunch, followed by an art session where we work with masks and words to try and express and make sense of some of the emotions, feelings and thoughts which the cancer has stirred up. This can help to stop things getting bottled up, reduce feelings of being out of control and stop teenagers feeling alone or different because of what's happening in their families.

Maggie's Centres also run information days for children aged 6-12 years who have a parent, carer or significant family member with cancer. They run on a few Saturdays a year, and again include a visit to the hospital where we get a chance to see behind the scenes, and understand a bit more about cancer treatments and how they are given. We find the hospital visit helps children to make sense of the things they might hear parents talking about at home.

The art session for the Kids' Day makes use of puppets, boxes and books to help us explore and express feelings.

During this day we run a session for parents while we are doing art with the kids, which allows families to meet others who are coping with the same issues. During this session we also try to help parents understand the ways that young children will cope when they feel scared or anxious.

Just like everybody else, when you don't understand what's happening you might get scared, and your imagination might begin to try and fill in the gaps. What we imagine is usually far worse than what is really happening, and so knowing the facts should help you feel more safe, and more in control. This is the main aim of the days we run for Teens and Children, but they will also help to normalise what's happening to your parent and to your family, and by meeting others who are dealing with the same issues you should feel less alone.

Visit Maggie's website:
www.maggiescentres.org

# Emma: The Special One

It was by chance I came across Emma's project when I stumbled upon her article in the Daily Record. What struck me was how young she was but her project was something that required maturity. It is not every day you come across a teenager who wants to inform other teenagers and not every teenager has a working enthusiasm needed to carry out such a demanding project. Emma is mature beyond her years and her energy to get things moving is as admirable as it is infectious. Her quest for knowledge and thirst to inform others about breast cancer is something I haven't came across in an adult, let alone a teenager.

I contacted Emma through her mum and things took off from there. I only wanted to let them know that there is support waiting for Emma's project and should they need any kind of assistance, I could provide some. Both Emma and Rosie are not the type of people who go about their business cap-in-hand; they want to do something in return when someone helps or donates to their cause. They are both remarkable citizens in the fund-raising world and an enormous credit to their cause. I have been as impressed as anyone in how they go about their work. They are incredibly industrious.

I used what I felt to be the main contacts that could help Emma with her project. I am fortunate to have these important contacts and within minutes Gina McKie from Scotland's largest radio station was quick to offer support. It wasn't long after when we all got to listen to Emma live on the radio.

Because of the nature of the book we needed someone to do the graphics and again, it didn't take too long before Leanne

Hamilton offered her time and skills as a graphic artist. Those two contacts were pinnacle and I will always be forever grateful to both Gina and Leanne.

As one phone call went to another and emails going back and forth, we found Emma's project going viral at an accelerated rate. For me, personally, one of the most interesting parts to this book is something that is often being asked: what has the mouse got to do with breast cancer?

A Cherokee Indian contact of mine read Emma's article and gave her the honourable tag name of Little Brave Mouse. I have often joked with Emma about the nick name and that she 'really looks like a mouse' and it does get laughs but in truth, her adopted Cherokee name is now sacred so she is stuck with it and it will follow her around with pride and honour. It is a lot to live up to but Emma has what it takes. She earned her name.

I am proud to say I have had the pleasure of spending quality time with great conversations with Emma. I know only too well what she has gone through so the need for calm and understanding was always first on my mind but we also shared some great laughs. It is hard to forget she is barely into her teens but we also can't forget that aside from the great serious work Emma does and for all what she, her sister Kate and mum Rosie, have had to endure, in the end Emma is a teenager and that can never be brushed aside.

I cannot thank Emma and Rosie enough for their trust in me. I learned so much about a subject that no-one is immune to.

I would also like to close by saying this one final thing…

Emma, you are one special young lady, truly unique and

amazingly special. You've gone through so much in the last year and I know you've cried like you could not imagine.

Times have been tough and life's circumstances have dealt you, Kate and mummy, a bad card. Your pain and anguish takes its toll on even the most hardened of adults but you kept going, you stayed strong, you kept up and you continued to briskly march through whatever was in front of you. You came out the other end, showing huge strength, courage and determination that I have never seen before in any walk of life.

You have produced a remarkable brand in your Eek! Project and the results that you have produced are simply extraordinary.

Many people have asked me how someone so young can go through all this and still manage to achieve all that you've achieved.

I tell them the same thing all the time…

It's because you are special.

Stephen Hamilton Nicol
~ Author ~

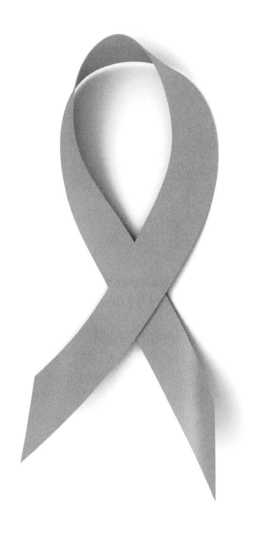

Visit Emma's website:
www.eekmymummy.co.uk

*Thank you all who have kindly donated and purchased*
*Eek! My Mummy Has Breast Cancer*

Emma Sutherland

For more information on
Breast Cancer Care Charity please visit:

www.nakedinspirations.co.uk

For more information on
Dot McQueen Photography please visit:

www.mcqphotography.co.uk

A Publication by SHN Publishing
www.shnpublishing.com

Lightning Source UK Ltd.
Milton Keynes UK
UKOW06f1029040813

214840UK00015B/39/P

9 781907 463785